Design: Judith Chant and Alison Lee

Recipe Photography: Peter Barry

Jacket and Illustration Artwork: Jane Winton, courtesy of

Bernard Thornton Artists, London

Editor: Josephine Bacon

CHARTWELL BOOKS
a division of Book Sales, Inc.
POST OFFICE BOX 7100
114 Northfield Avenue
Edison, NJ 08818-7100

CLB 4258

© 1995 CLB Publishing, Godalming, Surrey, U.K.

Printed and bound in Singapore
ISBN 0-7858-0289-4

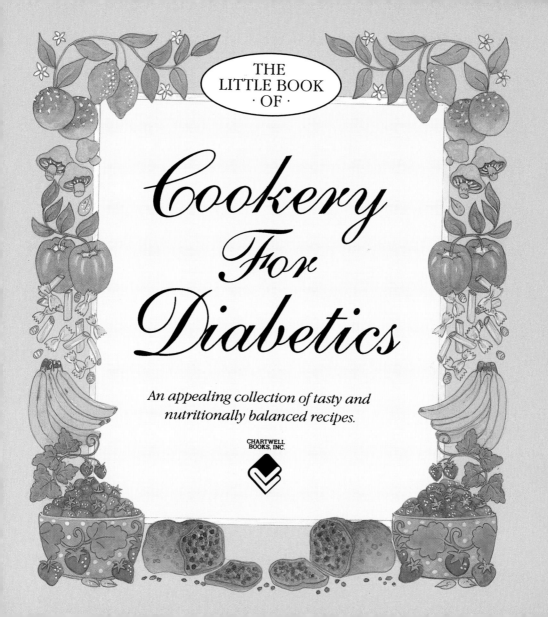

THE LITTLE BOOK · OF ·

Cookery For Diabetics

An appealing collection of tasty and nutritionally balanced recipes.

CHARTWELL BOOKS, INC.

Introduction

Eating the right foods is crucial to the health of all diabetics and a well planned approach to recipe planning is one of the keys to making delicious, well-balanced menus part of your everyday life.

This book is not intended as a guide book for diabetics, but simply as an extra source of carbohydrate and calorie counted recipes for diabetics who already know their dietary requirements and can confidently incorporate these recipes into their diet plan. There is no substitute for the the tailor-made advice which every diabetic should receive from a qualified dietitian when they are diagnosed.

Although individuals should be aware of their specific needs, there are a number of general guidelines which apply to the diabetic diet. Eating too much food at any one time should be avoided as it results in too much glucose for the system to cope with adequately. It is therefore advisable to have smallish meals and a variety of snacks throughout the day. This is particularly relevant to diabetics taking insulin, who should coincide their meals with the availability of insulin. Also important is the type of meal eaten. Those foods which are digested slowly further help to "spread" the release of glucose into the blood. Carbohydrate foods that contain a significant amount of dietary fiber or roughage are particularly important for this purpose as not only do they take longer to digest, but a high fiber diet helps to lower blood sugar levels. Finally, fat is another factor particularly relevant to diabetics. As diabetics are recommended to eat fiber-rich carbohydrate, a corresponding reduction in fat intake is often necessary if excess weight gain is to be avoided. Excess fat intake is also recognised as a major contributor to heart disease, and diabetics are already at a disadvantage as diabetes is recognised as a risk factor in developing such conditions.

The advice given to diabetics to follow a high-fiber, low-fat diet is advice that most people, diabetic or not, would be well advised to follow, and obviously as this pattern of eating becomes more commonplace so the range and availability of suitable ingredients increases. Hopefully, you will find some inspiring recipes in this little cookbook, and eventually gain the confidence to create your own. Obviously you will have to be very aware of your own particular dietary requirements but the following tips may also be of some help:

- When using artificial sweeteners ensure they are completely sugar-free
- Use whole-wheat flour wherever possible
- Use whole-wheat pasta and brown rice in place of their more refined cousins
- Fortify appropriate dishes such as soups and stews with pulses as they add valuable fiber
- Low-fat or reduced-fat cheeses should be used in place of full-fat cheeses
- Polyunsaturated oils such as sunflower, and polyunsaturated and mono-unsaturated margarines should be used
- All visible fat should be trimmed from chicken and meat
- Use low-fat yogurt in place of cream wherever possible

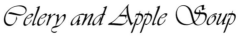

Celery and Apple Soup

SERVES 4

This unusual combination of ingredients produces a tasty soup, which is ideal as a first course or lunch dish when served with crusty whole-wheat rolls.

PREPARATION: 15 mins
COOKING: 45 mins
TOTAL CARBOHYDRATE: 60g PER SERVING: 15g
TOTAL ENERGY: 468 calories PER SERVING: 117 calories

---

2 tbsp polyunsaturated margarine
1 large onion, finely chopped
3 cooking apples, cored and sliced
5 cups vegetable broth
1 bay leaf
Salt and freshly ground black pepper
3 celery stalks, finely chopped
Finely sliced celery, to garnish

---

1. Melt the margarine in a large saucepan and stir in the onion. Fry gently for 5 minutes, or until the onion is soft but not browned.

2. Add the apple to the onion mixture and cook for a further 3 minutes, or until the apple begins to soften.

3. Stir half the broth into the onion and apple, along with the bay leaf and seasoning. Bring to a boil, cover, and simmer for 30 minutes. Remove the bay leaf.

4. Put the remaining broth into another pan along with the celery. Bring to a boil, then cover and simmer for 30 minutes.

5. Using a blender or food processor, blend the onion and apple mixture until smooth.

6. Whisk the pureed onion and apple mixture into the pan containing the broth and celery.

7. Return the pan to the heat and bring back to a boil. Serve immediately and garnish with the finely sliced celery.

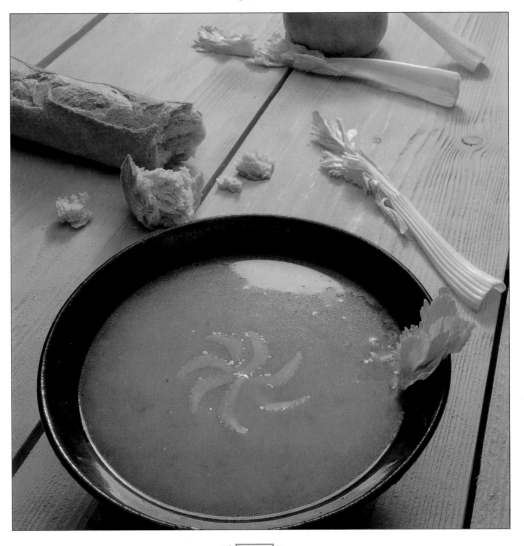

Salmon Pâté

SERVES 4

This highly nutritious, elegant paté is low in fat and very quick to prepare. Serve as a first course with a salad garnish, and accompany with melba toast or brown bread.

PREPARATION: 15 mins, plus chilling
TOTAL CARBOHYDRATE: 10g PER SERVING: negligible
TOTAL ENERGY: 669 calories PER SERVING: 167 calories

---

1 cup drained, canned salmon
½ cup low-fat cottage cheese
Few drops of lemon juice
Pinch of ground mace or nutmeg
¼ tsp Tabasco
Salt and freshly ground black pepper
2 tbsp 1% fat fromage blanc, or low-fat plain yogurt
4 small gherkin pickles

---

1. Remove the bones and skin, if any, from the salmon. Place the fish in the bowl of a food processor and process briefly to break it up.

2. Add the cottage cheese and process the machine in bursts, until the mixture is smooth.

3. Add the lemon juice, seasonings and fromage blanc, and process briefly until all the ingredients are well mixed.

4. Divide the mixture between 4 individual ramekins and smooth the surfaces. Refrigerate before serving.

5. Slit each gherkin lengthwise 4 or 5 times, making sure that you do not cut completely through the narrow end. Fan the gherkins out and use to garnish the top of the paté.

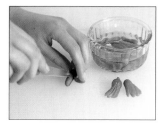

Step 5 Slice each gherkin lengthwise, 4 or 5 times, taking care not to cut right through the narrow end. Spread out into fan shapes.

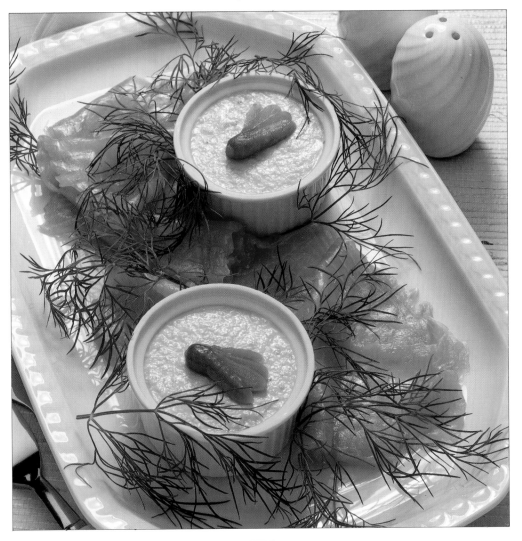

Pork with Green Peppers

SERVES 4

This quickly prepared stir-fried dish is ideal for a quick lunch or supper dish. Serve with brown rice or noodles.

PREPARATION: 15 mins
COOKING: 6 mins
TOTAL CARBOHYDRATE: 10g PER SERVING:
    negligible
TOTAL ENERGY: 930 calories PER SERVING:
    233 calories

1 lb pork tenderloin
2 tbsp sunflower oil
1 clove garlic, crushed
2 green bell peppers, cut into thin strips
1 tsp wine vinegar
2 tbsp chicken broth
1 tbsp Hoisin sauce
Salt and pepper
1 tsp cornstarch, mixed with a little water

1. Slice the pork thinly, then cut into narrow strips.

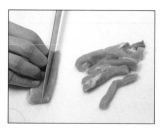

Step 1 Slice the pork thinly, then cut into narrow strips.

2. Heat the oil in a wok, add the garlic, green bell pepper, and the meat. Mix together well and stir-fry for 1 minute.

3. Stir in the vinegar, broth and Hoisin sauce. Season to taste and cook for a further 3 minutes.

4. Stir in the cornstarch mixture and cook, stirring constantly, until the sauce is thickened.

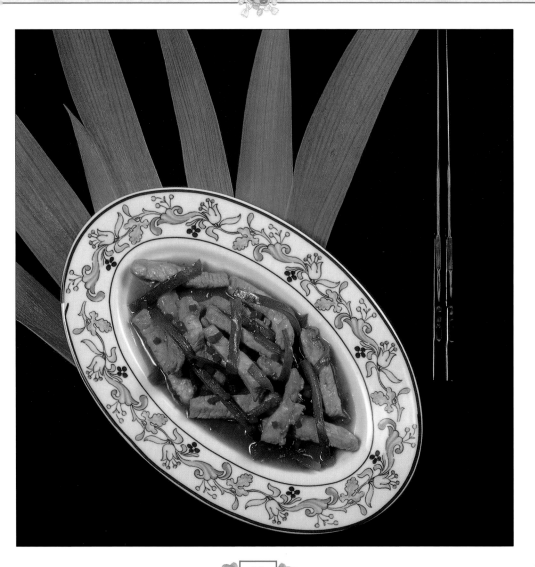

Chicken Stuffed Peppers

SERVES 6

Using chicken as a stuffing for peppers makes a lighter dish than the more usual meat stuffing. Serve either hot or cold, and accompany with rice and salad for a lunch or supper dish.

PREPARATION: 30 mins
COOKING: 45-50 mins
TOTAL CARBOHYDRATE: 160g PER SERVING: 30g
TOTAL ENERGY: 2704 calories PER SERVING:
    450 calories

3 large green or red bell peppers
2 tbsp polyunsaturated margarine
1 small onion, finely chopped
1 celery stalk, finely chopped
1 clove garlic, crushed
3 chicken breasts, skinned, boned and diced
2 tsp chopped parsley
Salt and freshly ground black pepper
½ loaf stale whole-wheat bread, made into
    crumbs
1-2 eggs, beaten
6 tsp dry brown breadcrumbs

1. Cut the bell peppers in half lengthwise and remove the cores and seeds. Leave the stems attached, if wished.

2. Melt the margarine in a skillet and add the onion, celery, garlic and chicken. Cook over a moderate heat until the vegetables are softened

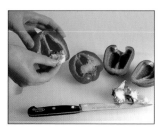

Step 1 Cut the peppers in half and remove the cores and seeds.

and the chicken is cooked. Add the parsley and season with salt and pepper.

3. Stir in the stale breadcrumbs and add enough beaten egg to make the mixture hold together.

4. Spoon the filling into each pepper half, mounding the top slightly. Place the peppers in a baking dish that holds them closely together.

5. Pour enough water around the peppers to come about ½-inch up their sides. Cover and bake in an oven preheated to 350°F, for about 45 minutes or until the peppers are just tender.

6. Sprinkle each pepper with the dried crumbs and place under a preheated broiler until golden brown.

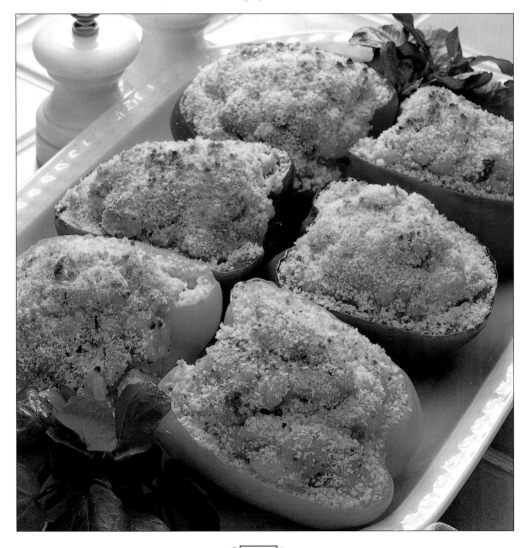

Fisherman's Stew

SERVES 6

This quick, economical and satisfying dish will please any fish fan. It makes an ideal meal for lunch or supper if served with brown rice, salad, or extra French bread.

PREPARATION: 20 mins
COOKING: 45 mins
TOTAL CARBOHYDRATE: 100g PER SERVING: 25g
TOTAL ENERGY: 2413 calories PER SERVING:
   403 calories

---

4 tbsp olive oil
2 large onions, sliced
1 red bell pepper, sliced
1⅓ cups sliced mushrooms
16-oz can tomatoes
Sprig dried thyme
Salt and freshly ground black pepper, to taste
Scant 2 cups water
2 lb firm, boneless white fish, skinned and cut
   into chunks
⅔ cup white wine or fish broth and wine
   mixed
2 tbsp chopped parsley
⅓ French stick, sliced and toasted

---

1. Heat the oil in a large saucepan, add the onions, and cook until beginning to look

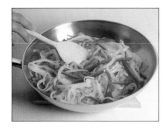

Step 1 Add the red pepper to the onions and cook until softened.

translucent. Add the red bell pepper and cook until softened.

2. Add the mushrooms and the tomatoes, and bring the mixture to a boil.

3. Add the thyme, seasoning and water, and simmer for 30 minutes.

4. Add the fish and wine, and cook for 10-15 minutes or until the fish is opaque and starts to flake. Carefully stir in the parsley.

5. To serve, place a piece of French bread in the bottom of each of 6 soup bowls and carefully spoon the stew over.

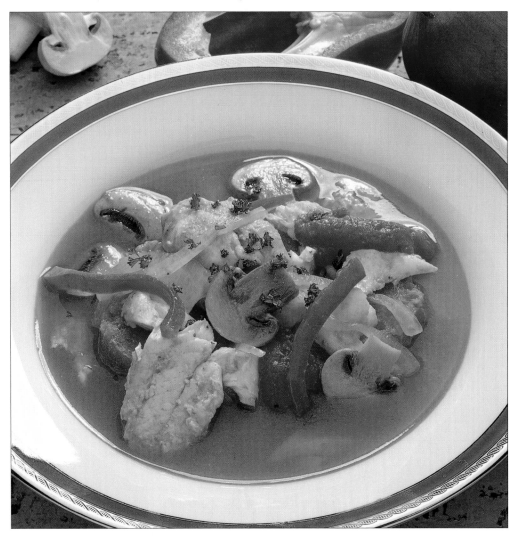

Savory Bean Pot

SERVES 4

Use canned kidney beans or other canned beans to make this dish easy and quick to prepare. Serve with whole-wheat pasta or brown rice.

PREPARATION: 20 mins
COOKING: 45 mins
TOTAL CARBOHYDRATE: 160g PER SERVING: 40g
TOTAL ENERGY: 1085 calories PER SERVING:
    271 calories

---

2 tbsp olive or sunflower oil
2 vegetable bouillon cubes, crumbled
2 medium onions
2 apples, grated
2 carrots, grated
3 tbsp tomato paste
1¼ cups water
2 tbsp white wine vinegar
1 tbsp mustard powder
1 tsp dried oregano
1 tsp ground cumin
Artificial sweetener equivalent to 2 tsp sugar
Salt and freshly ground black pepper
2 cups cooked red kidney beans
2 tbsp low-fat yogurt (optional)

---

1. Heat the oil in a nonstick pan. Add the crumbled bouillon cubes, onions, apples and carrots. Sauté for 5 minutes, stirring occasionally.

2. Mix the tomato paste with the water and add together with all the other ingredients except the beans and yogurt.

3. Stir the mixture well, cover, and simmer for 2 minutes.

4. Add the beans to the pan and stir in well, then transfer the mixture into a flameproof casserole.

5. Bake, covered, in an oven preheated to 350°F, for 35-40 minutes.

6. Look at the casserole after 20 minutes, and add a little more water if necessary. To serve, top with swirls of low-fat yogurt, if wished.

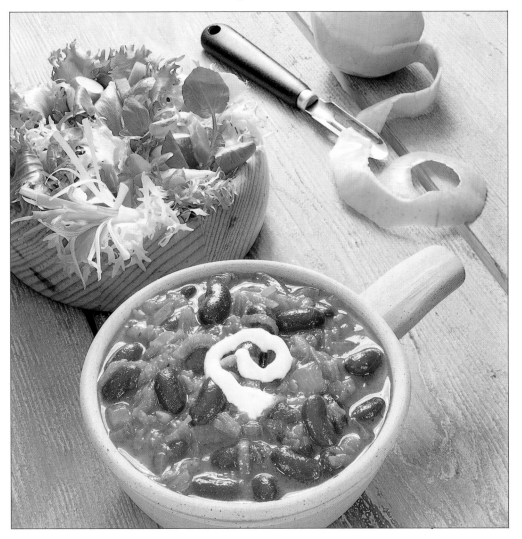

Sweet Pepper Steaks

SERVES 4

In this tasty dish, peppers, mustard and capers blend together to make a delicious spicy sauce for beef steak. Serve with either brown rice or jacket potatoes and broccoli.

PREPARATION: 30 mins, plus standing time
COOKING: 20 mins
TOTAL CARBOHYDRATE: 80g PER SERVING: 20g
TOTAL ENERGY: 1825 calories PER SERVING:
   456 calories

---

4 entrecôte steaks, about 4 oz each
2 cloves garlic, crushed
Freshly ground black pepper
3 tbsp olive or sunflower oil
2 shallots, finely chopped
4 tbsp capers
1⅓ cups sliced mushrooms
2 tbsp all-purpose flour
1¼ cups beef broth
4 tsp mustard
2 tsp Worcestershire sauce
½ cup white wine
2 tsp lemon juice
Pinch each dried thyme and rosemary
8 baby corn cobs, halved lengthwise
1 green bell pepper, sliced
1 red bell pepper, finely sliced
1 yellow bell pepper, finely sliced
4 tomatoes, skinned, seeded and cut into
   thin strips

---

1. Place the steaks on a chopping board and remove the excess fat. Rub both surfaces of each steak with the garlic and black pepper. Refrigerate for 30 minutes.

2. Heat the oil in a large skillet and quickly fry the steaks for 1 minute on each side. Remove the steaks from the pan and set aside.

3. Add the shallots, capers and mushrooms to the oil and meat juices in the skillet. Cook for about 1 minute.

4. Sprinkle the flour over the vegetables and fry gently until it begins to brown. Pour in the broth, stirring constantly. Add the mustard, Worcestershire sauce, wine, lemon juice and herbs as the sauce thickens.

5. Return the steaks to the sauce mixture, along with the baby corn, bell peppers and tomatoes. Simmer for 6-8 minutes, or until the steaks are cooked, but still pink in the center. Serve at once.

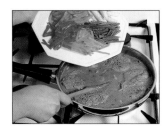

Step 5 Stir the corn, peppers and tomatoes into the sauce, mixing well to coat evenly.

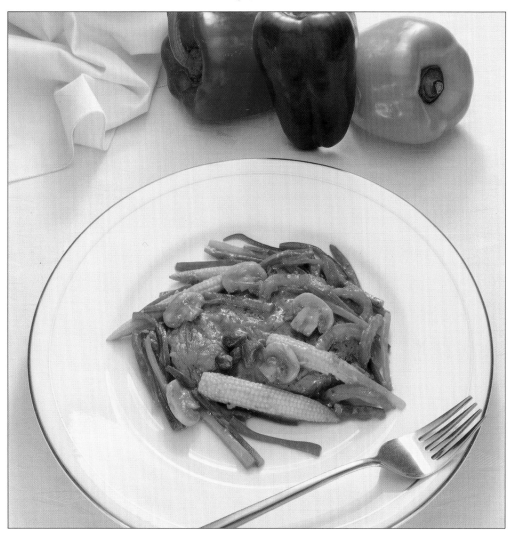

Farfalle with Tomato Sauce

SERVES 4

This is a great favorite with pasta fans – simple, delicious, and it looks good too!

PREPARATION: 10 mins
COOKING: 30 mins
TOTAL CARBOHYDRATE: 180g PER SERVING: 45g
TOTAL ENERGY: 2141 calories PER SERVING:
    310 calories

---

1 tbsp olive oil
2 cloves garlic, crushed
1 onion, sliced
½ tsp dried basil
2 × 14-oz cans chopped plum tomatoes
Salt and freshly ground black pepper
10 oz farfalle (pasta bows)
2 tbsp chopped fresh basil

---

1. Heat the oil in a deep saucepan. Add the garlic and onion and cook until softened. Add the dried basil and cook for 30 seconds.

2. Add the undrained tomatoes and season well. Bring to a boil, reduce the heat and simmer, uncovered, for about 20 minutes, or until the sauce is reduced by half.

3. Meanwhile, cook the pasta in a large saucepan of boiling, salted water for about 10

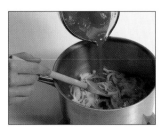

Step 3 Add the undrained tomatoes to the pan.

minutes or until "al dente." Rinse in hot water and drain well.

4. Push the sauce through a sieve, and stir in the fresh basil. Toss the sauce through the pasta and serve immediately.

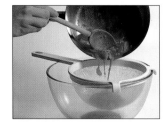

Step 4 Push the sauce through a sieve.

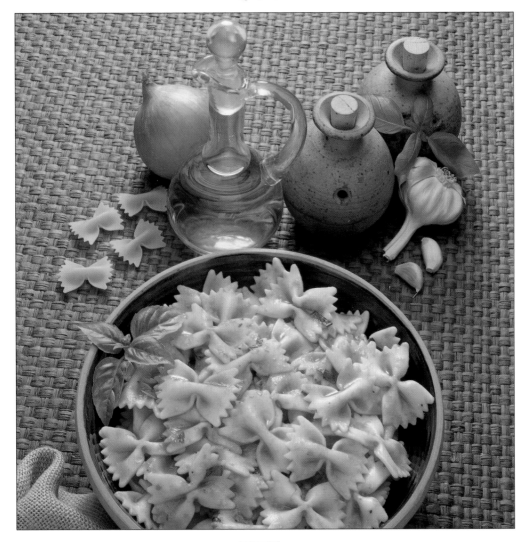

Poulet au Limon

SERVES 4

Roast chicken with a tang of lime makes an elegant yet quickly-made entree. Serve with salad and bread, or new potatoes and some vegetables.

PREPARATION: 25 mins, plus 4 hours marinating
COOKING: 35 mins
TOTAL CARBOHYDRATE: 10g PER SERVING: negligible
TOTAL ENERGY: 1581 calories PER SERVING: 395 calories

---

2 × 2 lb chickens
1 tsp basil
2 tbsp olive oil
4 limes
Salt and freshly ground black pepper
Artificial sweetener, to taste (optional)

---

1. Remove the leg ends and wing tips from the chickens.

2. Split each chicken in half lengthwise, cutting away the backbone completely and discarding it. Remove the skin.

3. Loosen the ball and socket joint in the leg and flatten each half of the chicken by hitting it with the flat side of a cleaver.

4. Season the chicken on both sides with salt and pepper and sprinkle over the basil. Place the chicken in a shallow dish and pour the oil over. Squeeze the juice from two of the limes and pour over the chicken. Cover and leave to

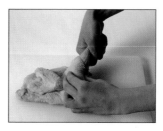

Step 3 Bend the chicken legs backward to loosen the ball and socket joints.

marinate in the refrigerator for 4 hours or overnight.

5. Transfer the chicken to a roasting pan and sprinkle with some of the marinade. Place in an oven preheated to 375°F, and roast for about 25 minutes, or until the juices run clear when pierced with a skewer. Baste the chicken occasionally with the marinade.

6. Cut off all the peel and pith from the remaining limes and slice them thinly. When the chicken is cooked, place the lime slices on top of the chicken and heat quickly under the broiler. Add a little sweetener to the limes, if wished.

7. Place the chicken in a serving dish and spoon over the cooking juices. Serve immediately.

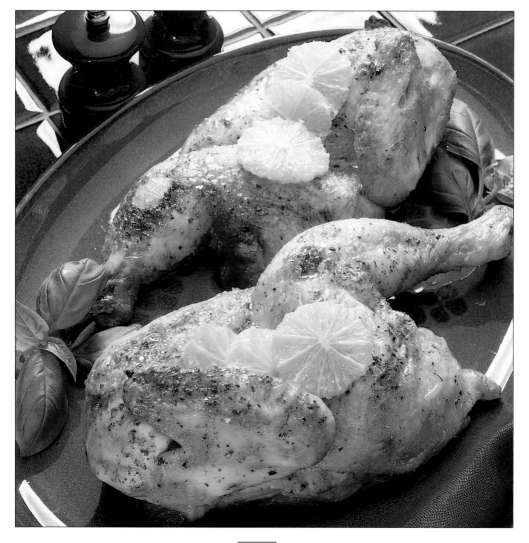

Andalusian Eggplant

SERVES 4

Tomatoes, rice and tuna fish are very popular ingredients in Spain, and they make a delicious stuffing for eggplant. Serve with a mixed salad, black olives and bread.

PREPARATION: 40 mins
COOKING: 50 mins
TOTAL CARBOHYDRATE: 70g PER SERVING: 20g
TOTAL ENERGY: 754 calories PER SERVING: 189 calories

4 small eggplants
2 tbsp olive oil
1 small onion, finely chopped
1 clove garlic, crushed
⅔ cup cooked brown rice
6½-oz can tuna in water, drained and flaked
1 tbsp low-fat plain yogurt
1 tsp curry powder
4 tomatoes, skinned, seeded and chopped
1 tbsp coarsely chopped parsley
Salt and freshly ground black pepper

1. Cut the eggplants in half lengthwise. Score the cut surfaces lightly with a sharp knife at regular intervals in a criss-cross pattern.

2. Brush the scored surfaces with 1 tbsp of the oil and place on a greased baking sheet.

3. Bake the eggplants in an oven preheated to 375°F, for 15 minutes or until beginning to soften.

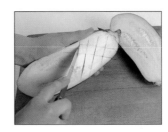

Step 1 Taking care not to break the skins, score the cut surfaces of the eggplant halves at regular intervals.

4. Cool the eggplants slightly, then carefully scoop out the center flesh from each half, taking care not to break the skins.

5. Sauté the onion gently in the remaining oil for 3 minutes, or until transparent.

6. Add the garlic and the eggplant flesh, and fry for a further 2 minutes.

7. Add the rice, tuna, yogurt, curry powder, tomatoes, parsley, and season to taste.

8. Mix the ingredients together well, then spoon equal amounts into the eggplant shells. Brush the eggplants with a little oil, return them to the oven on the baking sheet, and bake for a further 25 minutes.

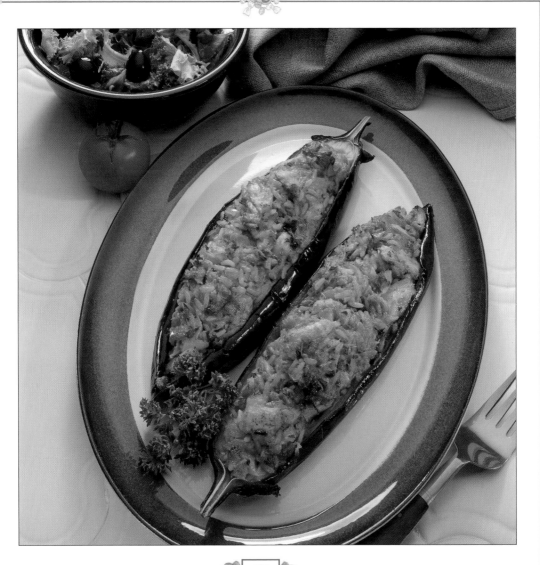

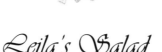

Leila's Salad

SERVES 4

This salad makes an ideal light lunch if served with crusty whole-wheat bread.

PREPARATION: 15 mins
COOKING: 30-35 mins
TOTAL CARBOHYDRATE: 130g PER SERVING: 35g
TOTAL ENERGY: 958 calories PER SERVING:
    240 calories

1½ cups long-grain brown rice
1 cup chopped pineapple
1 bunch scallions, finely chopped
½ cup slivered almonds, lightly toasted
½ bunch radishes, finely sliced
1 cup bean sprouts
Twists of lime, to garnish

Dressing
3 tbsp sunflower oil
1 tbsp sherry
Juice of 1 lime
1 tsp grated ginger root
Salt and freshly ground black pepper, to taste

---

1. Cook the rice in boiling, salted water for 30-35 minutes, or until tender. Drain and let cool.

2. Combine the rice with the pineapple, scallions, almonds, radishes and bean sprouts. If using fresh bean sprouts, blanch them in boiling water for 2 minutes, then refresh in cold water before using.

3. Mix all the dressing ingredients together in a bowl and whisk thoroughly with a fork until well blended.

4. Pour the dressing over the salad and fold in carefully. Refrigerate until required, then garnish with the lime twists.

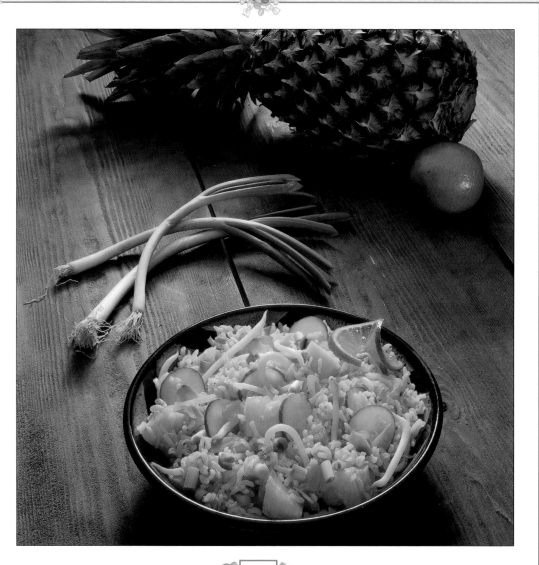

Zucchini Salad

SERVES 6

Raw vegetables are full of vitamins, and, although zucchini seems an unlikely vegetable to eat raw, it has a delicious flavor and texture. Serve this salad as an accompaniment to cold meat or poultry.

PREPARATION: 15 mins, plus 30 mins chilling
COOKING: 10 mins
TOTAL CARBOHYDRATE: 60g PER SERVING: 10g
TOTAL ENERGY: 1056 calories PER SERVING: 176 calories

---

2 cups whole-wheat macaroni
4 tomatoes
4-5 zucchini, thinly sliced
8 stuffed green olives, sliced
6 tbsp nonfat French dressing

---

1. Put the macaroni in a large saucepan and cover with plenty of boiling water. Add some salt and cook for 10-12 minutes, or until "al dente." Rinse in cold water and drain well.

2. Cut a small cross in the tops of the tomatoes and plunge into boiling water for about 30 seconds.

3. Drain them and cover with cold water, then remove the loosened skins using a sharp knife. Remove the cores and seeds of the tomatoes and coarsely chop the flesh.

4. Mix all the ingredients in a large bowl and refrigerate for 30 minutes before serving.

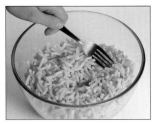

Step 1 Rinse the cooked macaroni in cold water, then drain well, forking it to prevent it sticking together.

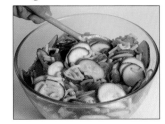

Step 4 Mix all the ingredients together well, stirring thoroughly to blend the dressing in evenly.

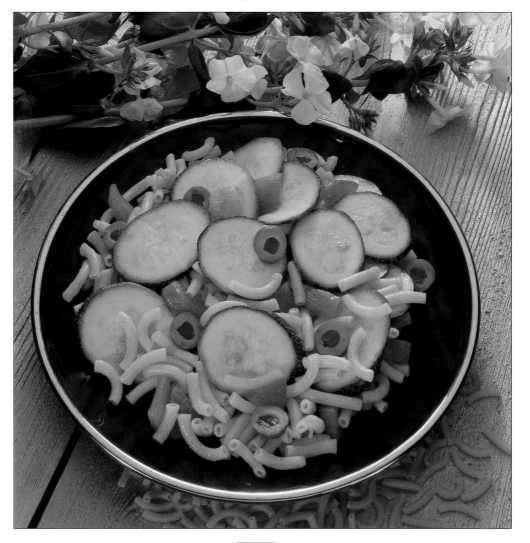

Flageolet Fiesta

SERVES 4

Serve this dish on its own as a first course or as a side dish. Red kidney beans can be used instead of the flageolet beans.

PREPARATION: 15 mins, plus 2 hours marinating
COOKING: 1 hour
TOTAL CARBOHYDRATE: 60g PER SERVING: 15g
TOTAL ENERGY: 865 calories   PER SERVING: 216
   calories

1¼ cups flageolet (green haricot) beans
1 medium onion
1 clove garlic
1 cucumber
2 tbsp chopped parsley
2 tbsp chopped mint
2 tbsp olive oil
Juice and grated peel of 1 lemon
Salt and freshly ground black pepper
Watercress, to garnish

---

1. Put the cooked beans in a mixing bowl.

2. Peel and finely chop the onion.

3. Crush the garlic and chop the cucumber into bite-sized pieces.

4. Add the onion, garlic, cucumber, herbs, oil, lemon juice and peel to the beans and mix well.

5. Add seasoning to taste and leave to marinate for 2 hours.

6. Transfer to a clean serving dish and garnish with watercress before serving.

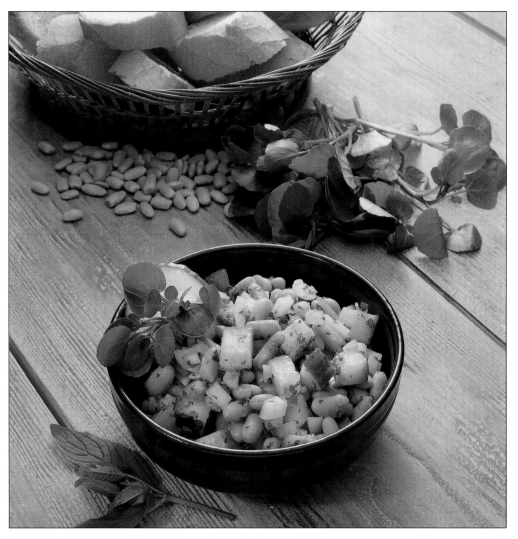

Strawberry Cloud

SERVES 4-6

Tofu blended with strawberries makes a tasty, quick and healthy dessert that is ideal for summer. Other fruit, such as apricots, peaches, mangoes or pitted cherries, would taste equally delicious.

PREPARATION: 10 mins
TOTAL CARBOHYDRATE: 30g PER SERVING: 10g
TOTAL ENERGY: 372 calories PER SERVING: 93
   calories

1 lb strawberries
1 × 10-oz pack silken tofu
Juice of ½ lemon
Artificial sweetener, to taste
Few drops vanilla extract

1. Wash and hull the strawberries. Reserve a few for decoration, then roughly chop the rest.

2. Drain the tofu and put into a blender or food processor, together with the strawberries and lemon juice. Liquidize until smooth.

3. Add the liquid sweetener and vanilla extract to taste, mixing in well.

4. Divide the mixture between 4-6 individual serving dishes and decorate with the reserved strawberries. Refrigerate until required.

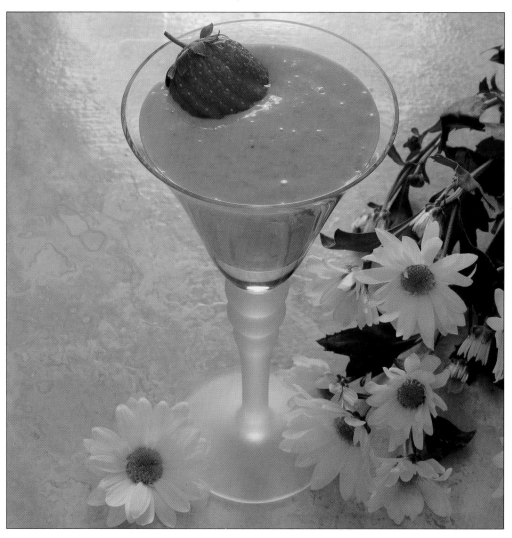

Almond-Stuffed Figs

SERVES 4

Fresh figs are often available from major supermarkets and good produce markets, but if unavailable fresh peach halves would work equally well.

PREPARATION: 20 mins
TOTAL CARBOHYDRATE: 60g PER SERVING: 15g
TOTAL ENERGY: 560 calories PER SERVING: 140
    calories

4 large ripe figs
4 tbsp ground almonds
2 tbsp orange juice
2 tbsp finely chopped dried apricots
4 tbsp low-fat plain yogurt
Finely grated peel of ½ orange
Wedges of fig and mint or strawberry leaves, to
    decorate

1. Cut each fig into quarters, taking care not to cut right down through the base.

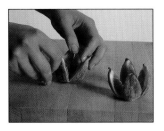

Step 2 Ease the four sections of each fig outward, to form a flower shape.

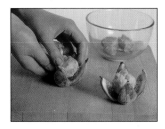

Step 4 Divide the almond mixture evenly between the four figs, and press it into the center of each one.

2. Ease the four sections of each fig outward to form a flower shape.

3. Put the ground almonds, orange juice and chopped apricots into a small bowl and mix together thoroughly.

4. Divide the mixture into four, and press it into the center of each fig.

5. For the sauce, mix together the yogurt and orange zest, then thin it down slightly with a little water or more orange juice.

6. Spoon a small pool of orange yogurt onto each of four serving plates, and place a stuffed fig in the center of each pool. Decorate with the additional wedges of fig and the mint or strawberry leaves.

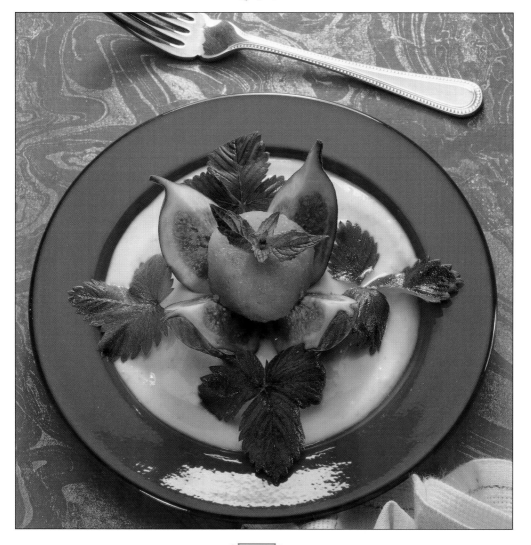

Baked Bananas Sauce à La Poire

SERVES 4

Baked bananas are an established favorite dessert, and served with this delightful fruity sauce they are particularly delicious.

PREPARATION: 10 mins
COOKING: 10 mins
TOTAL CARBOHYDRATE: 100g PER SERVING: 25g
TOTAL ENERGY: 422 calories PER SERVING: 105 calories

2 small oranges
2 ripe pears, peeled and cored
Artificial sweetener, to taste
2 bananas

1. Using a potato peeler, pare the peel from one of the oranges, taking care not to include too much white pith.

2. Cut the orange peel into very thin strips with a sharp knife, and blanch in boiling water for 2-3 minutes, to soften. Drain and set aside.

3. Peel and segment one orange and squeeze the juice from the other.

4. Place the orange juice and pears in a food processor. Puree until smooth. Sweeten to taste.

5. Peel the bananas and halve them lengthwise. Place in a flameproof dish and pour the pear puree over the top. Cover and bake in an oven preheated to 350°F, for 10 minutes or until the bananas are soft.

6. Decorate with orange segments and strips of orange peel. Serve immediately.

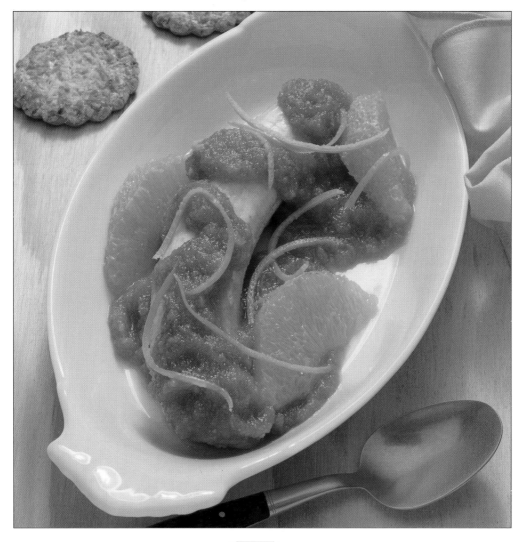

Apple Spice Ring

SERVES 10

This delicious and healthy cake can be served hot as a dessert with apple sauce.

PREPARATION: 15 mins
COOKING: 45 mins
TOTAL CARBOHYDRATE: 170g   PER SERVING: 20g
TOTAL ENERGY: 1588 calories   PER SERVING:
   159 calories

---

1 lb dessert apples, cored
¾ cup ground hazelnuts
1 cup whole-wheat flour
2 tbsp bran
1½ tsp baking powder
1 tsp ground cinnamon
Pinch of ground nutmeg
Pinch of ground cardamom
2 tbsp polyunsaturated margarine
8 tbsp skim milk
Apple slices, to decorate

---

1. Grate the apples on the coarse side of a grater.

2. Place in a mixing bowl along with the hazelnuts.

3. Stir in the flour, bran, baking powder and spices. Mix to blend well.

4. Add the margarine and beat until it is evenly blended.

5. Stir in the milk and mix to a stiff batter.

6. Carefully spoon into a greased 8-inch ring mold and level the top.

7. Bake in an oven preheated to 350°F, for 45 minutes or until a skewer inserted into the center of the cake comes out clean.

8. Let cool slightly in the mold, then transfer to a rack to cool.

9. Decorate with apple slices just before serving.

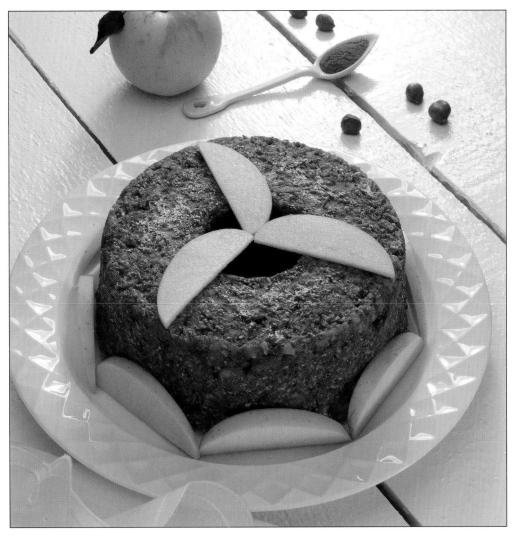

Fruit Loaf

MAKES 2 loaves, each loaf makes 18 slices

Use any combination of your favorite dried fruits in this recipe for a variation. It is worth making two loaves since they will freeze for up to two months if wrapped in foil.

PREPARATION: about 2 hours
COOKING: 35-40 mins
TOTAL CARBOHYDRATE: 320g (per loaf) PER
    SLICE: 20g
TOTAL ENERGY: 1557 calories (per loaf) PER
    SLICE: 87 calories

3¼ cups whole-wheat bread flour
½ tsp cinnamon
½ tsp nutmeg
½ tsp salt
1 cup golden raisins
1 cup sun-dried raisins
¼ cup cut mixed citrus peel
1 package of fast-rising yeast
2 tbsp sunflower oil
About 1¼ cups lukewarm skim milk
1 large egg

---

1. Put the flour, spices and salt into a large mixing bowl. Stir in the dried fruit and peel, mixing well to distribute it evenly.

2. Sprinkle over the yeast, and mix this directly into the dry ingredients.

3. Put the oil, milk and egg into a large bowl and beat together with a fork until the egg is broken up evenly. Add the mixture to the flour and mix together, stirring until the batter becomes soft and elastic.

4. Turn the dough onto a lightly floured work surface, and knead for about 10 minutes or until smooth.

5. Return the dough to the bowl and cover with a damp cloth or a piece of plastic wrap. Let rise in a warm place for about 1 hour or until doubled in size.

6. Knock the dough back to remove the air, and turn it out onto the surface again. Knead the dough for about 5 minutes, then cut it in two.

7. Shape each piece of dough to fit 2 × 7-inch nonstick loaf pans. Cover each loaf as before and leave in a warm place until doubled in size.

8. Bake in an oven preheated to 400°F, for 35-40 minutes, removing them after 20 minutes to brush the tops with a little milk to glaze. The loaves are cooked when they sound hollow when tapped on the bottom.

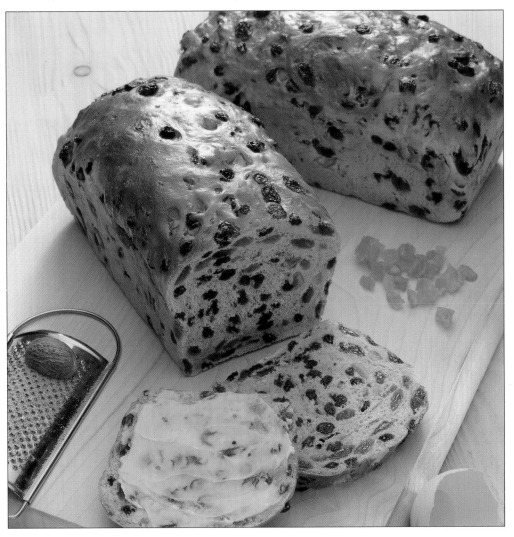

Index

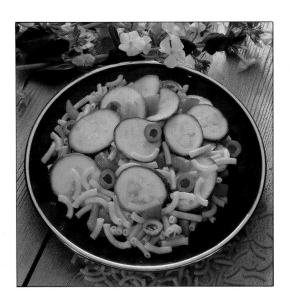